# WAS THIS PERSON MURDERED?

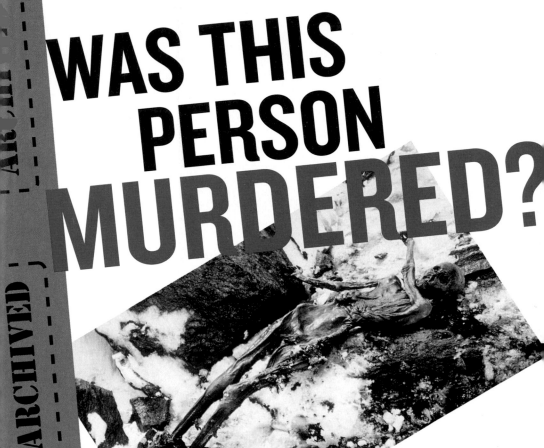

Hikers in the mountains of Austria and Italy stumbled across this body in 1991. Immediately, they called the police. When the police arrived, they suspected that the man had been murdered. Were they correct?

# MAYBE!

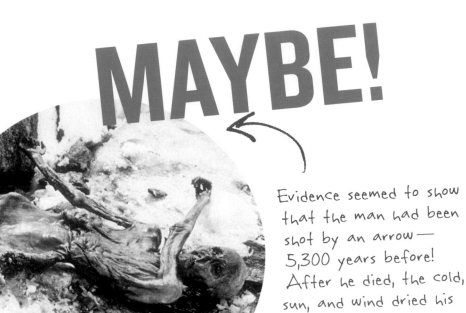

Evidence seemed to show that the man had been shot by an arrow — 5,300 years before! After he died, the cold, sun, and wind dried his body. Then a glacier covered him, creating a natural mummy that's now called Ötzi the Iceman!

Book design Red Herring Design/NYC

Library of Congress Cataloging-in-Publication Data
Grace, N. B.
Mummies unwrapped! : the science of mummy-making /
By N. B. Grace.
p. cm. – (24/7: science behind the scenes)
Includes bibliographical references and index.
ISBN-13: 978-0-531-12076-7 (lib. bdg.)   978-0-531-17533-0 (pbk.)
ISBN-10: 0-531-12076-7 (lib. bdg.)  0-531-17533-2 (pbk.)
1. Mummies—Juvenile literature. 2. Embalming—Juvenile literature. I. Title.
GN293.G73 2006
363.3—dc22    2006021238

© 2008 Scholastic Inc.
All right reserved. Published by Franklin Watts, an imprint of Scholastic Inc.

Published simultaneously in Canada. Printed in China.  62

SCHOLASTIC, FRANKLIN WATTS, and associated logos are trademarks and/or registered trademarks of Scholastic Inc.
6 7 8 9 10  R  17 16 15 14 13

# MUMMIES
# UNWRAPPED!

## The Science
## of Mummy-Making

N. B. Grace

**WARNING:** This book shows how bodies are preserved, either by people or by nature. Dead bodies can be gruesome! Mummy photos can be gross. If that freaks you out, read something else!

**Franklin Watts**
An imprint of Scholastic Inc.
New York • Toronto • London • Auckland • Sydney
Mexico City • New Delhi • Hong Kong
Danbury, Connecticut

# CONTENTS

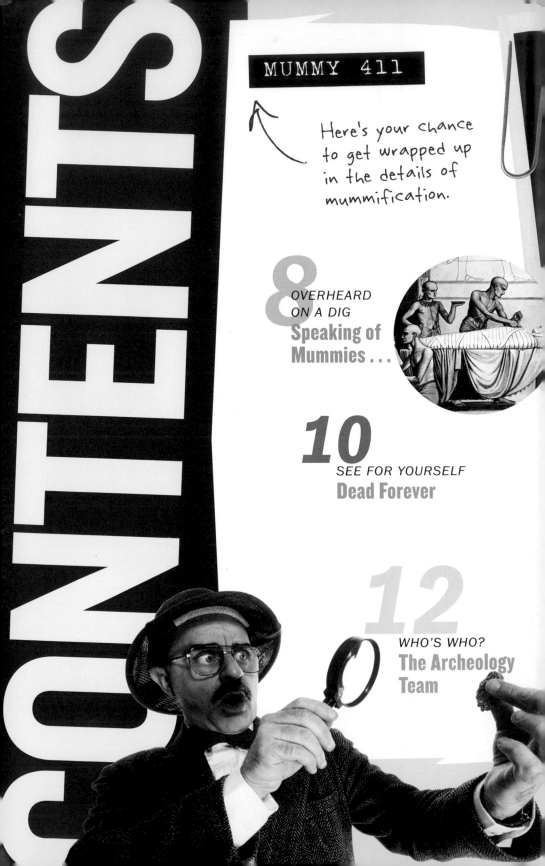

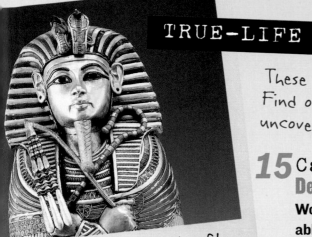

These stories are 100% real. Find out how archeologists uncovered these mysteries.

King Tut of Egypt left incredible treasures behind.

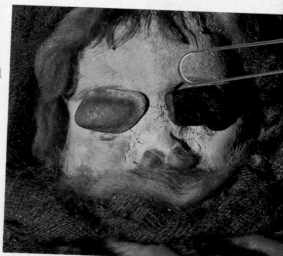

Mysterious people in China made this mummy from a baby.

This mummy was murdered in Denmark—over 2,000 years ago.

5

# MUMMY DOWNLOAD

Here's even more amazing stuff about mummies for you to unwrap.

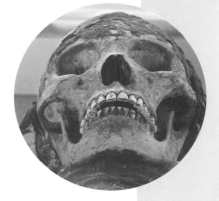

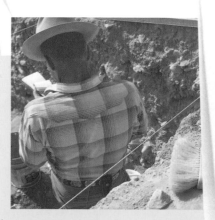

## YELLOW PAGES

A body is found. It's thousands of years old.

Maybe it had been wrapped in strips of cloth and buried in a tomb. Maybe it had been frozen in a glacier. Possibly it had been preserved in a marshy bog.

## MUMMY 411

Whatever form a mummy takes, it can say a lot. It's an archeologist's job to find out what this corpse has to tell about the civilization from which it came.

IN THIS SECTION:

▶ how archeologists really talk;

▶ how ancient Egyptians made mummies;

▶ and who's on the team that looks for and examines mummies.

# Speaking of Mummies...

**Archeologists have their own way of talking. Find out what their vocabulary means.**

Professor, do you ever wish you were an **archeologist** in Egypt about a hundred years ago?

Definitely. That's when there was still a good **mummy** or two lying around. You know about the **tomb** at Deir el Bahri, right?

**archeologist**
(ar-kee-OL-uh-jist) a person who studies past ways of life

**mummy**
(MUH-mee) a dead body that has been preserved and has lasted a very long time

**tomb**
(toom) a grave or room for holding a dead body. In Egypt, tombs were often dug into the side of cliffs.

Of course. That's the tomb found in the 1800s, with about 50 mummies inside. They weren't too **decayed**, either.

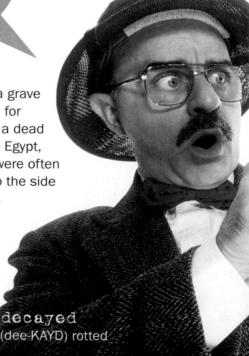

**decayed**
(dee-KAYD) rotted

Lots of stuff had been stolen, though. Those Egyptian **embalmers** were good at **preserving** bodies. But the security wasn't so tight.

**embalmers**
(em-BAWL-murz) people who embalm, or treat a corpse so that it won't decay

**preserving**
(prih-ZURV-ing) protecting something so that it doesn't change or decay

Keep digging, Professor. Maybe we'll find an ancient **artifact** everyone else has overlooked.

**artifact**
(ART-uh-fakt) an object, such as a tool, weapon, or ornament made by human beings

# Say What?

**Here's some other lingo archeologists might use on the job.**

**bog dog**
(bawg dawg) the preserved body of a dog found in bogs in northern Europe, near where human bog bodies have been found
*"We didn't find any human bog bodies, but there was a well-preserved bog dog out there."*

**mummy gape**
(MUH-mee gayp) Mummies often have woven straps around their heads to hold their jaws closed. If that strap is loosened, the mouth falls open, which makes the mummy look surprised. (*Gape* means staring with your mouth open.)
*"The mummy was well preserved, but it had a bad case of mummy gape."*

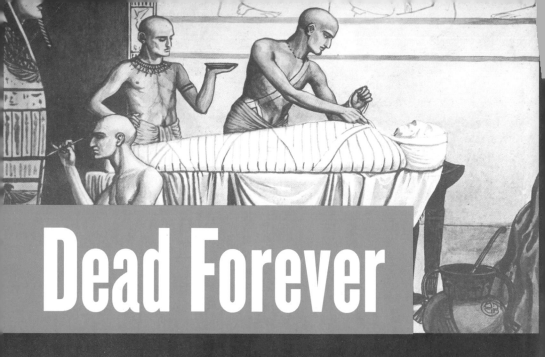

# Dead Forever

## The Egyptians made mummies that were built to last. How did they do it?

You'd be amazed at how quickly a dead body starts to decay and turn into mush. Not long after death, disease-carrying cells called **bacteria** in the intestines start to digest other organs. Chemicals in other cells also start to break down **tissues** inside the body.

What's more, blowflies and other insects lay eggs on wounds and body openings. Those eggs will hatch into maggots looking for their next meal.

Eventually, there's nothing left but a skeleton.

### Look, No Decay!

The ancient Egyptians made a discovery. When they buried their dead in the hot, dry sands of the desert, the bodies didn't decay.

The Egyptians didn't know that bacteria need moisture to attack tissues. But they noticed that if they kept **corpses** dry, they'd last longer. Starting about 2600 BC, Egyptians also observed that if they removed the moist brain and organs inside the bodies, those corpses would last even longer.

And according to the Egyptians, these life-like bodies could later join the person's spirit in the afterlife.

Egyptian embalmers probably didn't leave instructions. But here are some of the steps they may have included if they had recorded the 70-day process of creating a mummy.

# MAKING A MUMMY

**Step #1** Make an **incision** on the left side of the corpse's body. Take out the moist organs that will cause the body to decay—including the lungs, liver, stomach, and intestines. Leave the heart in the body. (The ancient Egyptians believed that the heart was the center of thought and emotion.)

**Step #2** Dry the organs. Wrap them in linen. Then place them in containers called **canopic jars**. (These jars often had stoppers that may have been intended to look like the heads of the dead people.)

**Step #3** Insert an iron rod into the nose. Push it upward through the skull bone and into the brain cavity. Drain the brain out through the nose.

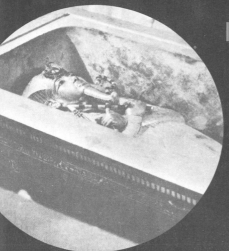

**Step #4** Place the body in a bed of **natron**. (Natron is a mixture of salt and a substance like baking soda.) It's good for drying the body. Once the body is dry, wash it and cover it with oils and spices.

**Step #5** Stuff the body of the corpse to give it a human shape. Stitch up the incision. You may also decorate the body with colored dyes, makeup, and jewelry.

**King Tut's mummy with a gold mask.**

**Step #6** Cover the entire body in **resin**—sticky stuff that will keep the body from falling apart. Wrap the body with linen strips. You may need up to 450 square yards (375 sq m). Place **amulets** (jewelry with religious meaning) on the body to protect it from curses.

**Step #7** Cover the head with a mask that looks like the person who was mummified.

11

# The Archeology Team

**Archeologists often work with other experts to uncover the secrets of mummies and their tombs.**

### PATHOLOGISTS
They're experts in human disease. They may study mummies to find evidence of diseases.

### FIELD ASSISTANTS
They help archeologists on digs by carefully sifting through dirt to find buried artifacts, measuring and mapping the site, and recording the finds.

### ARCHEOLOGISTS
They're scientists who study artifacts from past civilizations to learn how ancient people lived.

### MUMMIES!
Mummies can tell researchers about the health issues of past peoples, how long they lived, what they ate, and more. Art and artifacts in tombs can give information about everyday life.

### TEXTILE EXPERTS
They examine the mummies' clothes and wrappings.

### FORENSIC ARTISTS
They use their knowledge of the human face to re-create mummies' faces.

### RADIOLOGISTS
They're experts in X-rays and other technologies that create images of bodies and internal organs. X-rays and CT scans of mummies can reveal broken bones, as well as artifacts hidden in the wrappings.

### ANTHROPOLOGISTS
They're scientists who study the biology, customs, and beliefs of humans both in the past and the present.

# TRUE-LIFE
# CASE FILES!

**24 hours a day, 7 days a week, 365 days a year, archeologists are digging up mysteries.**

IN THIS SECTION:

▶ what the experts learned about the most famous mummy of all time;

▶ how some surprising mummies showed up in China;

▶ and a theory about why a man found in a bog was murdered 2,000 years ago!

# A Guide to Mummies

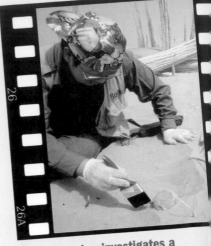

A worker investigates a site in China, where salt mummies were found.

**Not all mummies were created by Egyptian embalmers. Some are 100% natural.**

Egyptian embalmers had the basic idea. They kept their corpses clean, dry, and covered. That way, bacteria wouldn't make the corpses decay. And insects wouldn't attack them, either.

Other bodies have become mummies by accident. Here's how.

**Extreme cold:** You met Ötzi the Iceman on page 1. His body was frozen under a **glacier**. The extreme cold kept bacteria from attacking his body.

In 1972, eight more ice mummies were found in Greenland. The winter wind and the dry cold had sucked the moisture out of the bodies.

**Dry heat:** Preserved bodies have been found in the deserts of China, Chile, Peru, and Egypt. The weather dries the bodies out before they can rot.

**Salt:** Salt can preserve bodies by removing the moisture. Five mummies were found in a salt mine in Iran between 1993 and 2005. One had died 1,700 years before, possibly in a cave-in.

**Bogs:** Bogs are soft, waterlogged areas of ground. Mummies have been found in bogs of England, Germany, and Scandinavia. Bogs contain plants that create chemicals that preserve bodies.

Valley of the Kings,
Egypt
1922

# Desperately Seeking Tut

**Would archeologists be able
to find the mummy of this
young Egyptian king?**

# Searching for King Tut

**Archeologist Howard Carter is searching for the mummy of King Tutankhamen, the young king.**

In the Egyptian desert lies a mysterious place called the Valley of the Kings. This is where the kings of ancient Egypt were buried about 3,000 years ago.

More than a hundred years ago, archeologists began digging up the remains of these kings—or **pharaohs**, as they were called. By then, most of the tombs had been robbed. But archeologists did find many treasures, such as gold and jewelry, as well as mummies.

In 1917, a British archeologist named Howard Carter began looking for a mummy that had never been found—that of King Tutankhamen.

Carter and other archeologists knew little about Tutankhamen. From artifacts found in other tombs, they knew that he had ruled Egypt for only about nine years, from 1361 to 1352 BC. They also knew that he had married a girl named Ankhesenpaaten, the daughter of the previous king.

Beyond that, Tut's life was a mystery. No one knew who Tut's mother or father had been. Or what kind of ruler he had been. Or why he had died so young. Carter hoped that the king's tomb would provide some answers.

British archeologist Howard Carter was determined to find the tomb of King Tutankhamen. The graves of the major pharaohs had all been robbed. But King Tut was less well known. Carter hoped that his tomb would still be intact.

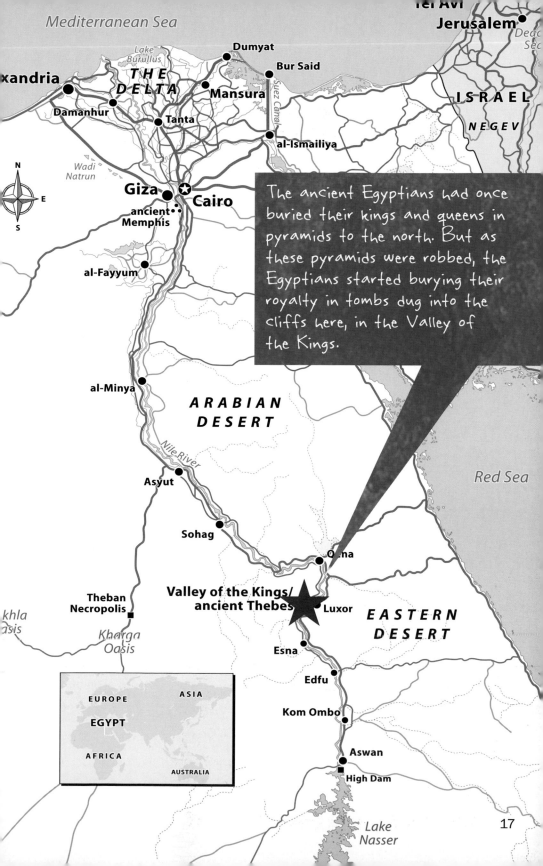

Mediterranean Sea

Lake Burullus

THE DELTA

xandria
Damanhur
Tanta
Dumyat
Bur Said
Mansura
al-Ismailiya

ISRAEL

Tel Aviv
Jerusalem
Dead Sea

NEGEV

Suez Canal

N
W E
S

Wadi Natrun

Giza
Cairo
ancient Memphis

al-Fayyum

al-Minya

ARABIAN DESERT

Nile River

Asyut

Sohag

Red Sea

Qena

Theban Necropolis

Valley of the Kings/ ancient Thebes

Luxor

EASTERN DESERT

khla asis

Kharga Oasis

Esna

Edfu

Kom Ombo

EUROPE
ASIA
EGYPT
AFRICA
AUSTRALIA

Aswan
High Dam

Lake Nasser

The ancient Egyptians had once buried their kings and queens in pyramids to the north. But as these pyramids were robbed, the Egyptians started burying their royalty in tombs dug into the cliffs here, in the Valley of the Kings.

Carter also hoped that Tut's tomb would give information about Egyptian burial practices. No modern explorers had ever found a mummy in its original tomb, with the original artifacts. Only one mummy, Amenophis II, had been found in his tomb. But all the artifacts buried with him had been stolen.

Backed by a wealthy man named Lord Carnarvon, Carter searched for Tut's tomb for five years. During that time, the men became close friends. But they found no trace of Tut.

# The Secret Staircase

**Carter gets one last chance to find Tut's mummy.**

By the summer of 1922, Lord Carnarvon was ready to give up. He told his friend Howard Carter that he would no longer fund the expedition. He had already spent a fortune—for nothing.

Carter begged Carnarvon. He reminded him that there was still one area that they had not yet explored. It was a small plot near the entrance to the tomb of Ramses VI. They had avoided the area because that tomb was so popular with tourists.

Carnarvon agreed to just one more year of

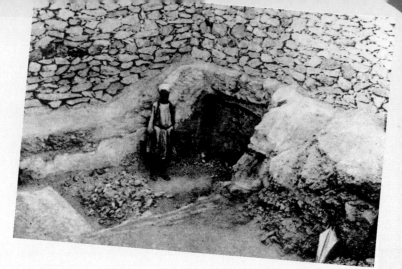

An Egyptian worker stands in front of the door to Tut's tomb. At the top of this door is a seal showing that someone royal had been buried within.

exploration. On November 1, Carter and his team began to work.

A few days later, on November 4, a young boy brought water for the workers. He cleared a space on the ground so that he could put down his water jars. That's when he saw a step cut into the rock!

Carter told his men to start digging. They found 11 more steps that led down to a door. Near the top of the door, Carter saw an official seal. It showed that someone royal had been buried there.

Carter then asked his workmen to replace the sand so that no one could see that there was a tomb below.

Immediately, Carter sent a telegram to Lord Carnarvon in England. "At last we have made wonderful discovery in the Valley," Carter wrote. "A magnificent tomb with seals intact; re-covered same for your arrival; congratulations."

What would Carter and his team find inside the tomb? Carter would wait until his friend arrived.

# Exploring the Tomb

**Carter and Carnarvon enter the tomb—and find "wonderful things."**

It took three weeks for Lord Carnarvon to arrive from England. Carter then ordered his workmen to clear away the sand and rubble blocking the stairs and the entrance to the tomb.

When they did, they immediately spotted the official seal of Tutankhamen near the bottom of the door.

They knew they had found what they were looking for.

The team moved farther into the tomb and came to a second doorway. It was sealed with bricks. Carter removed some of the bricks and stuck a candle through the hole. He peered into the room beyond.

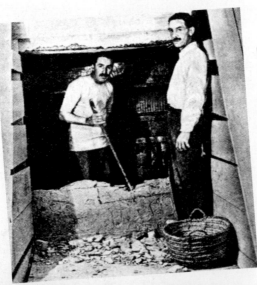

Howard Carter (*left*) stands with his assistant, A. R. Callender, at the entrance to the tomb. Inside, they'd find about 5,000 artifacts.

There was a long silence.

"Can you see anything?" Lord Carnarvon asked.

"Yes, wonderful things!" Carter answered.

Carter was looking into the first room of Tut's tomb. It was filled with treasures: life-sized statues, a chariot, furniture, gold. Lots of gold.

In December, Carter and his team started the huge job of emptying the room. They photographed every object. They recorded where everything had been placed. Then they carefully wrapped each object to keep it safe. And finally, everything was moved to the Egyptian Museum in Cairo, the capital of Egypt.

In February 1923, Carter and Lord Carnarvon invited a special group to see King Tut's tomb. At the end of the day, one reporter wrote, "This has perhaps been the most extraordinary day in the whole history of Egyptian **excavation**."

The guests saw treasures from the tomb, as well as artwork on the walls. Carter also opened the door to the burial chamber—and saw what seemed to be a wall of pure gold.

Carter would learn later that it was a shrine built to protect the stone

It took months for Carter and his team to carefully remove the contents of the first room. He then was able to open a door leading into another room. He saw a huge, gold shrine built to protect King Tut's stone sarcophagus.

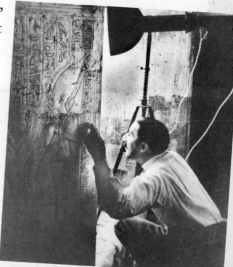

**sarcophagus**, or coffin, of King Tutankhamen.

A few months later, Lord Carnarvon died of an infected mosquito bite. The press turned this natural event into something more exciting: "The Curse of Tutankhamen." Shortly after that, Carter had to close the tomb while he and Carnarvon's family fought with the Egyptian government over the right to examine it.

After a long year of waiting, Carter was finally able to return to his work. It was then that he opened the sarcophagus and found a second coffin.

Inside that was a third coffin made of solid gold. It was covered with sticky resin, a substance made from the sap of plants and trees.

When that coffin was opened, Carter saw the body of King Tut for the first time. It was covered with strips of cloth coated with resin. The mummy was wearing a gold mask with the youthful face of King Tutankhamen.

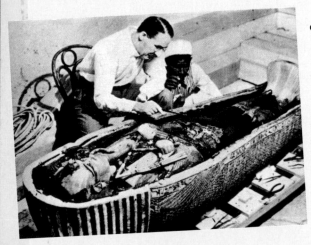

Howard Carter and an Egyptian worker examine one of King Tut's coffins. The mummy of King Tut had been placed inside three nested, mummy-shaped coffins. Two of these coffins were painted gold, and one was made of solid gold.

# Unwrapping King Tut's Secrets

**Scientists examine King Tut's mummy for clues about life in ancient Egypt.**

In November 1925, Carter and his team began to examine King Tut's mummy. First, they unwrapped all the strips of cloth and took note of all the jewelry and religious objects that were wrapped with the body.

Unfortunately, they weren't so careful with the body itself. They cut off the head to examine it. Then they cut the mask away from the skull with hot knives. They took off the mummy's pelvis, arms, and legs.

They put all the parts on a large tray. Two **forensic** scientists examined them. They studied King Tut's bones and teeth and decided that he had been between 18 and 22 when he died.

Tut's mummy, like other Egyptian mummies, also told archeologists a lot about Egyptian religious beliefs. Ancient Egyptians believed that corpses would need their bodies in the afterlife. That's why it was important to preserve them.

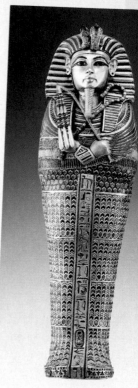

This is the innermost coffin (*above*) in King Tutankhamen's tomb. The coffin was made of almost 250 pounds (113 kg) of gold and covered in valuable stones. Inside this coffin was Tut's mummy.

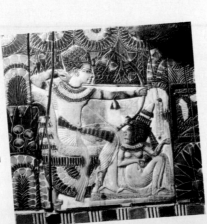

The walls of King Tut's tombs are covered in murals showing scenes from his life. Here, Tut's wife, Ankhesenamun, appears next to him on a hunting expedition.

That's also why the tombs were equipped with everything that the dead person would need for a happy afterlife. Tut's tomb was packed with furniture, games, food, and jewelry. There were even little statues called *shabtis* that were supposed to work as servants in the afterlife.

Carter and his team did have one disappointment. There were no written records that could answer questions about Tut's background and his reign.

In 1926, Carter rewrapped the mummy, put it back in the sarcophagus in the tomb, and laid a glass lid on top. That's where King Tut lay, undisturbed, for the next 40 years.

# FLUFFY, THE MUMMY

**Not all mummies were human.**

Ancient Egyptians didn't just mummify humans. They also made mummies out of animals.

Sometimes, they mummified animals that were **dedicated** to a god or goddess. For example, archeologists have found animal cemeteries in Egypt that were filled with thousands of mummies of cats, hawks, ibises (a type of bird), and crocodiles.

They also mummified the pets of people who had just died. That way, the deceased would be able to play with her pet in the afterlife!

A cat mummy, carefully painted.

# Up Close and Personal with Tut

**In 1968, more scientists take a look at Tut—and discover a possible murder mystery.**

In 1968, a new team of investigators got permission to x-ray King Tutankhamen's body.

The investigators weren't allowed to move the mummy. So they had to roll an old, portable X-ray machine into the tomb. Still, they made a surprising discovery. The X-ray showed that there were bone fragments in Tut's skull.

Had someone hit King Tut in the head and murdered him?

Some experts argue that the young king had been murdered. Others say that the bone fragments aren't proof of a murder. They could have resulted from the embalming process—or when Carter and his team were roughly examining the body.

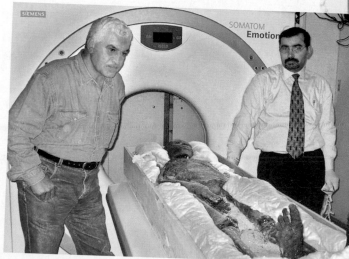

In 2005, scientists performed a CT scan on King Tut. CT scans can create 3D Images of the inside of bodies. Here, Zahi Hawass (*left*), from the Egyptian government, stands next to the 3,300-year-old mummy as it enters the CT machine.

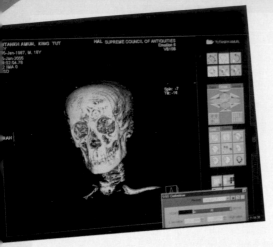

Even after the 2005 CT scan of Tut's skull (*shown here*), the mystery of the king's death was not solved.

Then, in 2005, researchers were allowed to do a **CT scan** of the mummy. Scientists said that this test proved that the king had *not* been hit in the head.

So how did Tut die? The CT scan also showed that the king had a badly broken leg. Could he have died from an infection resulting from this break? Or maybe it was poisoning. . . .

One thing's for certain. The discovery of King Tut's mummy and tomb was one of the most important discoveries in the history of **archeology**. It has solved many mysteries about ancient Egypt.

And there are probably still more mysteries to be unwrapped. . . . **24/7**

**[Mummy Fact]**
One quote in a tomb read, "O flesh of the king, do not decay, do not rot, do not stink."

*In the next case, investigators are astonished to find some mummies that seem very far from home!*

# The Puzzling Case of the Mummies in China

These mummies were tall,
fair-skinned—and European.
So how did they end up
in China?

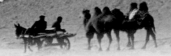

# "He Looked Like My Brother Dave!"

## What are these mummies of ancient Europeans doing in China?

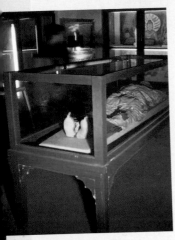

In 1988, Dr. Victor Mair took a group of students to a museum in a remote part of China called Urumchi. He spotted a sign pointing to a back room, "Mummies Exhibit." There, he found the mummies shown here.

The room in the museum in Urumchi, China was dimly lit. But with a flashlight, Dr. Victor Mair could see the bodies in the display cases. And what he saw amazed him.

They were ancient mummies found in China. But they looked like **Caucasians**—white Europeans.

One mummy was about 6'6" (198 cm), with reddish-brown hair. Dr. Mair couldn't stop staring at him. "He looked like my brother Dave sleeping there, and that's what really got me," he reported later.

The mummy wore striped leggings, white knee-high boots, and a two-piece suit. He was surrounded by ten hats, including a beret and a hat made of white felt that looked like a helmet.

Another mummy was a woman wearing a long red robe and deerskin boots. She had designs painted on her face. Red yarn was threaded through her ear lobes.

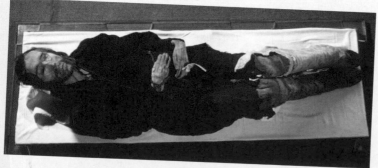

This is the mummy that looked like Dr. Mair's brother Dave. This mummy is 6'6", (198 cm) with reddish-brown hair—and extremely colorful leggings.

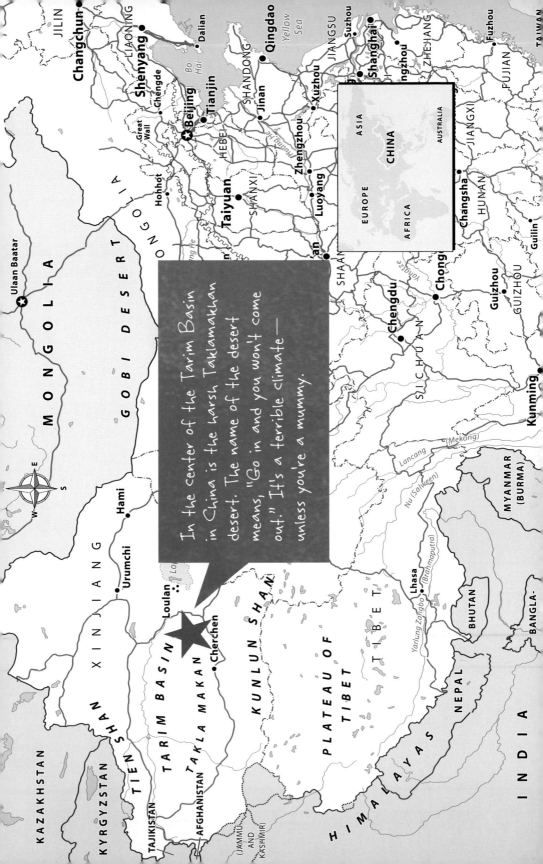

In the center of the Tarim Basin in China is the harsh Taklamakan desert. The name of the desert means, "Go in and you won't come out." It's a terrible climate— unless you're a mummy.

# JUST ADD SALT

## How did these ancient people preserve their dead?

The mummy-makers of the Tarim Basin had preserved their dead by burying them in tombs in the salt beds of the Tarim Basin. Salt is a "moisture hog," says archeologist Elizabeth Barber. It soaked up all the moisture in the bodies.

What's more, desert air is extremely dry. This also helped dry out the bodies. Without moisture, bacteria couldn't grow.

Unlike the Egyptians, the ancient people of the Tarim Basin didn't remove the mummies' internal organs. Still, the salt and the hot, dry air had preserved the bodies and the clothing and objects with which they were buried.

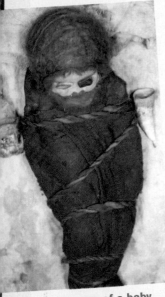

This mummy of a baby girl was buried with a baby bottle. Her mother may have died. Survivors may have tried to keep her alive by bottle-feeding her.

There were two other women as well, along with a baby girl. The child had been carefully bundled up in a blanket. Small blue stones covered her eyes. There was a blue cap on her head. Bits of red wool were stuffed in her nostrils.

The group looked almost as if they were sleeping. But they were mummies—and they had died centuries before.

More than a hundred mummies have been found in the deserts of western China. Some were discovered in the late 1800s. Many were found in the 1970s, when roads and pipes were being laid in the area.

Dr. Mair returned home to the U.S. But he couldn't forget about the Caucasian mummies.

# Where Are You From?

**The mummies start to tell their stories.**

The mummies hadn't said a word. But Dr. Mair, a professor of Chinese language and literature, realized that they could completely retell world history.

Most scholars believed that the first time Europeans and Chinese met was 2,000 years ago when the Silk Road was established. The Silk Road was a major trading route between Europe and Asia.

But Dr. Mair had suspected that Europeans had come to China much earlier. There were many ancient stories about mysterious people in western China. These people were said to be quite tall, with blond or reddish hair, blue or green eyes, and light skin.

The mummies of the Tarim Basin seemed to indicate that these old stories could have been true. Scientists used a technique called **carbon dating** to figure out the age of these bodies. The mummies were about 3,000 years old. So instead of Europeans and Asians first meeting 2,000 years ago, they could have met 1,000 or more years before that!

For more information about carbon dating see "How Old Is It?" on page 51.

# Clues from the Grave

## What other stories do the mummies have to tell?

In 1996, Dr. Mair gathered a team of experts to examine the mummies more closely. The team included an archeologist, a forensic anthropologist, and a textile expert. They traveled to China to examine the mummies and their clothes.

The team studied a facial reconstruction of one of the mummies. Artists create reconstructions of faces when police or archeologists find a skull and want to know what that person looked like. In this case, the facial reconstruction seemed to support Dr. Mair's theory. The mummy's face looked European.

An expert in textiles, Elizabeth Barber, also examined the clothes buried with the mummies.

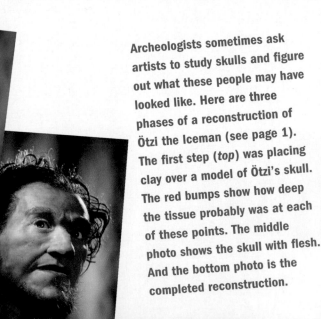

Archeologists sometimes ask artists to study skulls and figure out what these people may have looked like. Here are three phases of a reconstruction of Ötzi the Iceman (see page 1). The first step (*top*) was placing clay over a model of Ötzi's skull. The red bumps show how deep the tissue probably was at each of these points. The middle photo shows the skull with flesh. And the bottom photo is the completed reconstruction.

She was stunned by the colorful fabric woven in a plaid pattern. This pattern looked very similar to one used by Celtic people in northern Europe. Were these fabrics clues to where the mummy people may have come from?

There were seashells found with some of the mummies as well. This was surprising, since the western China desert is so far from the ocean! At the time, these seashells, called **cowries**, were used as money. So the fact that they were in the tombs may have meant that the mummy people traded with other groups of people.

The experts considered other clues as well. On top of the male mummy's grave, mourners had buried a dead horse and saddle. Perhaps it was thought that he would need them in the afterlife. To Dr. Mair, that meant that horses were important to these ancient people. Perhaps they had even traveled by horse from Europe.

And then came another convincing piece of evidence. Dr. Mair and the others climbed a steep cliff and entered a cave. On the walls they found paintings of people with light hair and blue eyes—people who looked a lot like the mummies from the Tarim Basin! The art looked a lot like ancient artwork from Europe.

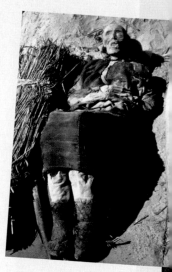

This mummy of a woman was also found in Tarim Basin. Like many of the mummies found in this area, she was wearing brightly colored, woven clothing. She was also buried with a stack of sticks. Was this firewood to keep her warm in the afterlife?

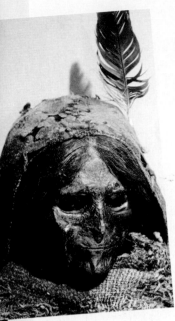

This mummy of a young woman is called the "Beauty of Loulan." She was carefully buried in a wool wrap, a leather skirt, fur and leather moccasins—and a wool hat decorated with a feather.

But it wasn't until 2006 that Dr. Mair got the solid evidence he had been looking for. He was able to examine some of the mummies' **DNA**.

DNA is information that's stored in almost every cell of your body. It's a kind of code that describes almost everything about you—your hair color, the length of your toes, and even what diseases you may develop. People who are related have similar DNA. So a DNA test of the mummies would tell Dr. Mair to whom these ancient people were most likely to be related.

And almost 20 years after Dr. Mair first saw the mummies in Urumchi, the DNA evidence seemed to confirm his theory. The mummies seemed to be related to Europeans. They were Caucasian. Dr. Mair wrote, "The new finds are . . . forcing a re-examination of old Chinese books that describe . . . legendary figures of great height, with deep-set blue or green eyes, long noses, full beards, and red or blond hair."

These old stories, Dr. Mair concluded, now seem to be have been fact. **24/7**

What would you think if you found a body with a noose around its neck? That foul play is involved, of course. Find out about a 2,000-year-old murder mystery in the bogs of northern Europe.

Tollund, Denmark
1950

# The Mystery of the Bog Bodies

Another body is found in a marshy bog in Denmark. And this one was murdered. Why?

# Murdered Mummy

**Two brothers get quite a shock one day as they work in a bog.**

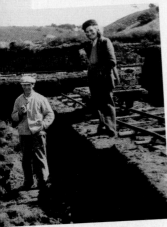

Viggo and Grethe Hojgaard stand in the peat bog where the Tollund Man was discovered.

It probably started off as just another day for brothers Emil and Viggo Hojgaard. They were working in a bog in the village of Tollund, in Denmark.

Bogs are soft, waterlogged areas of ground. They can be dark and eerie. Over the centuries, many legends have been written about them. People used to believe that trolls and spirits lived there, awaiting innocent travelers.

In fact, bogs *can* be dangerous places. People can lose their footing, get sucked into the ooze, and drown.

Sometimes people are even killed and their bodies thrown into the bog!

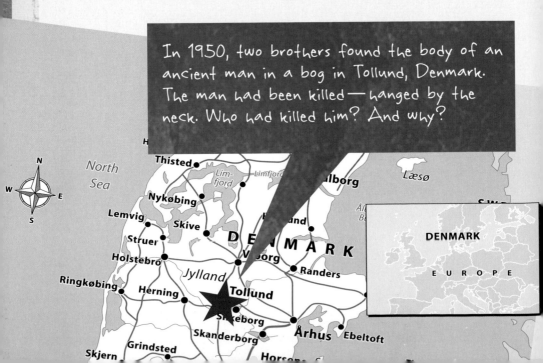

In 1950, two brothers found the body of an ancient man in a bog in Tollund, Denmark. The man had been killed — hanged by the neck. Who had killed him? And why?

North Sea

Thisted

Lim-fjord — Limfjord

Ålborg

Læsø

Nykøbing

Lemvig

Skive

DENMARK

Struer

Holstebro

Viborg

Jylland

Randers

Ringkøbing

Herning

Tollund

Silkeborg

Skanderborg

Århus

Ebeltoft

Skjern

Grindsted

Horsens

DENMARK

EUROPE

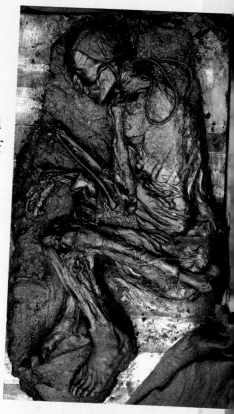

On that day in 1950, the Hojgaard brothers had been cutting **peat**, a type of dense soil made from rotted plants. They had to dig into the ground with shovels and then cut the peat into bricks. These bricks would then be dried and burned for fuel.

Suddenly, they saw something shocking: a man's face! The brothers uncovered the rest of the body. They found a small man with a well-preserved face. He looked as if he were sleeping. But there was one clue that this man hadn't just fallen asleep in the bog and drowned. It was the rope tied around his neck.

The Hojgaard brothers were sure that they had stumbled upon a murder victim. They called the police.

When the police arrived, they took one look at the body and called the local museum. Two ancient bodies had been found in the bog before. The police suspected that this was not a recent murder.

They were right. Scientists discovered that the Tollund Man, as he is now called, had been killed about 2,000 years before. Now they just had to figure out why.

This mummy, called the Tollund Man, was found in a bog in Denmark in 1950. The 2,000-year-old mummy was carefully dug out of the bog, placed in a box, and taken to a museum.

# BOGGED DOWN
## Bogs can preserve bodies for thousands of years.

Why don't bodies left in bogs decay? Scientists think there are three main reasons.

▶ Running water collects oxygen molecules, which help plants, fish, and bacteria live. But bog water is very still. That means that it doesn't contain much oxygen. And that means that it's hard for the organisms that feed on bodies to live there.

▶ Bogs also contain a kind of acid released by plants. This acid preserves bodies much as vinegar preserves pickles.

▶ Many bogs contain **sphagnum**, a kind of moss. This moss produces a chemical called tannin. This is the same chemical used to tan animal skins. When a body is put in a bog, the tannin preserves the flesh and turns it a deep, dark brown.

# Tollund Man Speaks
## Scientists try to find out how Tollund Man lived and died.

Bog bodies have been discovered in England, Wales, Ireland, Denmark, the Netherlands, and Germany since the 1600s. They are rare compared to Egyptian mummies. Millions of mummies were made in Egypt. Only a few hundred bog mummies have been found in the past 400 years.

The Tollund Man is the best-preserved bog mummy ever discovered. He's also the first bog mummy to be examined by scientists. He was examined in 1950; more recently, in 2002, scientists did a CT scan of his body to learn even more.

Here's what scientists discovered about Tollund Man.

- He died around 350 BC.
- His wisdom teeth had come in—so he was at least 20 years old. Scientists think that he was probably about 40.
- He was 5'3" (160 cm) tall, although his body could have shrunk in the bog.
- He had scars on his feet that showed that he walked barefoot some of the time.
- His last meal was soup. And there was barley in the soup with fungus on it that can cause hallucinations. Some scientists think that this was added to the meal to make him unconscious before he was killed.

Experts in Denmark examine the head of the Tollund Man with an endoscope. That's a long, thin instrument with a camera on the end. They found that the Tollund Man's brain was very well preserved.

The mummy's head was removed from the body in 1950. It was considered impossible to save the entire body.

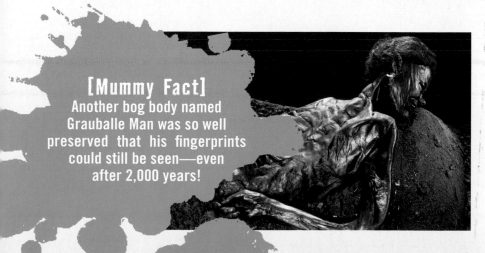

**[Mummy Fact]**
Another bog body named Grauballe Man was so well preserved that his fingerprints could still be seen—even after 2,000 years!

# Same Facts, Different Theories
## Was the Tollund Man killed as a religious sacrifice?

But why was the Tollund Man killed? Scientists agree that he was murdered. But why? Was he the victim of a crime? Or was he punished for some crime?

Or was there another reason?

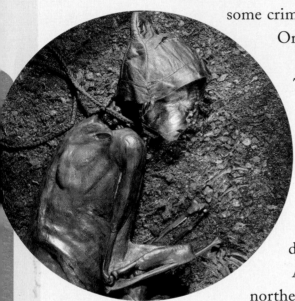

The Tollund Man seems to have been gently placed in the bog after he was hanged. Was he killed as part of some religious sacrifice?

Some experts believe that the Tollund Man may have been a religious sacrifice. People who lived in this area at the time of his death didn't leave written records. But Romans traveled to these lands, and they wrote down what they had learned during their travels.

According to these accounts, northern Europeans sometimes offered human sacrifices to their gods and goddesses. Perhaps they wanted to ask for a good harvest or the return of warm weather.

These experts point out that the Tollund Man was not treated as a criminal. His body wasn't carelessly thrown into the bog. Instead, he was placed gently in a grave dug into the peat. He was laid on his side, with his legs bent against his stomach. What's more, scientists think that his eyelids and mouth were closed after death.

Did the people in what is now Tollund, Denmark, practice human sacrifice? Scientists can't say for certain. They will continue to examine the bog bodies as new technologies are invented.

Unfortunately, in the case of the Tollund Man, the old saying is true: Dead men *don't* tell tales. 24/7

**[Bog Mummy Fact]**
Bog bodies have also been found in the marshes of the southeastern United States. These bodies of Native Americans are about 8,000 years old. Most of them died of natural causes.

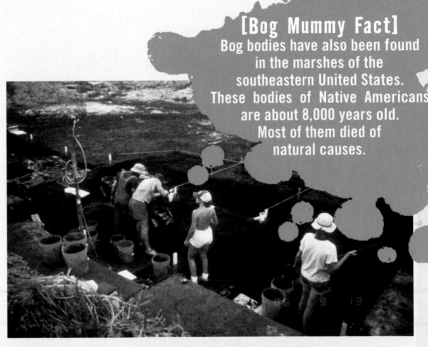

In 1982, a backhoe operator discovered human remains in this peat bog near Titusville, Florida. Over the next few years, researchers from Florida State University found the remains of 167 figures. Carbon dating indicated that these people had been buried at least 7,000 years before.

# BOG WOMAN

## The Tollund Man wasn't the first mysterious mummy found in a bog in Denmark.

It was 12 years before the discovery of the Tollund Man. And it was only 260 feet (80 m) from where that mummy would later be discovered.

A farmer in Denmark was digging for peat when his shovel struck a body.

This mummy is known as the Elling Woman. Her body was not as well preserved as that of the Tollund Man. Still, experts were able to determine that she too had been hanged. And like the Tollund Man, she had been buried with care. She had been placed on her side in a grave in the peat. And a blanket had been wrapped around her feet.

Was the Elling Woman another human sacrifice?

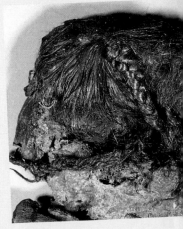

The so-called Elling Woman was found in 1938, just 260 feet (80 m) from where the Tollund Man would be found 12 years later.

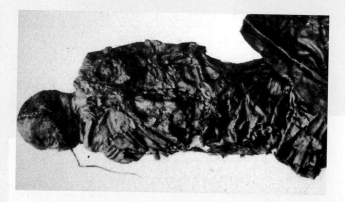

# MUMMY
## DOWNLOAD

**Here's some other info about mummies—dug up just for you!**

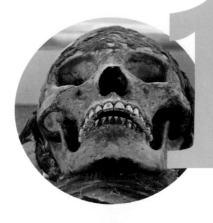

**5000–2000 BC**
**First Mummies Made**
The Chinchorro people begin making mummies in the area along the coast of what is now Peru and Chile. These are the oldest human-made mummies ever found. They are re-discovered by an archeologist in the early 1900s.

# Key Dates in the History of

**Humans have tried to preserve the bodies of their dead for thousands of years.**

**3300 BC The Ice Man Freezes Over**
Ötzi the Iceman (*below*), one of the most amazing natural mummies ever found, dies in the Alps. He is re-discovered in 1991. His grass cape, bow and arrows, shoes, and other items have all been preserved.

**3000 BC Walk Like an Egyptian**
The Egyptians start making mummies. Around 2600 BC, they start removing the corpses' organs to prevent the bodies from rotting.

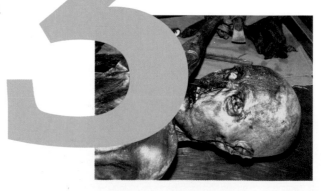

### 1352 BC **A Young King Dies**

King Tutankhamen (*below*) dies in Egypt; his body is mummified. His tomb and mummy are re-discovered in 1922.

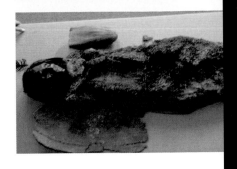

*See Case #1.*

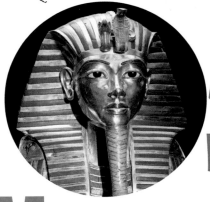

### 1000 BC **Mystery Mummies in China!**

Colorfully dressed mummies like the one above are buried in tombs in the Tarim Basin in China. Their bodies have been preserved by the salt surrounding them, as well as by the dry desert air. The mummies are re-discovered starting in the late 1800s.

*See Case #2.*

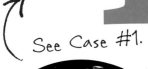

# Mummy-Making

### AD 1475 **Mummies in North America**

Six women and two children are buried in a tomb in what is now Greenland. It's likely that the people who buried them did not intend to mummify them. However, the dry cold preserved their bodies. These mummies were re-discovered in 1972.

### 350 BC **Murder in Denmark**

A man is killed—probably as part of a religious **ritual**—in what is now Denmark. His body is thrown in a bog and becomes a mummy (*below right*). The Tollund Man, as he is called, is found in 1950.

*See Case #3.*

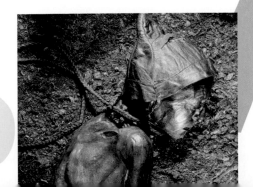

# In the News

# The Case of the Mummy's Tooth

CAIRO, EGYPT—June 2007

The mummy of one of Egypt's few female pharaohs has finally been identified.

Hatshepsut came to power in the 15th century BC, when her husband, Tuthmosis II died. Originally, she said she was filling in for her young son until he was old enough to rule. But seven years later, she had herself declared king.

Yes, *king*. Traditionally, the head of Egypt was a man. So Hatshepsut had herself depicted in artwork with a beard and men's clothing. And she was often referred to as "his majesty." King Hatshepsut ruled Egypt for 22 years.

After Hatshepsut's death, the next pharaoh tried to erase her from history. Scholars thought they had found her mummy in 1903, but they but couldn't be sure. All identifying markings on the mummy had long been removed.

But recently, archeologists did a CT scan of a wooden box that was known to belong to Hatshepsut. Inside the box was a tooth. And it matched exactly a hole in the jaw of the 1903 mummy. "We therefore have scientific proof that this is the mummy of Queen Hatshepsut," said researcher Dr. Zahi Hawass.

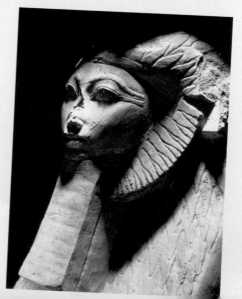

**King Hatshepsut ordered artists to depict her as a man with a beard in murals and sculptures.**

# Tattooed Woman Warrior Found in Peru

TRUJILLO, PERU—May 2006

A well-preserved mummy of a young woman with very elaborate tattoos covering her arms, legs, and feet has been found in Peru. The tattoos included images of spiders as well as pictures of imaginary creatures.

"It was as if she was wrapped up yesterday—no information has been lost," anthropologist John Verano told *National Geographic*.

The mummy was found in a pyramid made of mud brick. The body had been wrapped in hundreds of layers of cloth strips.

The woman, who lived around 450 BC, was also buried with sewing needles, weaving tools, and jewelry. Her tomb also included two huge war clubs and 23 tools used for throwing spears. "The war clubs are clear symbols not only of combat but of power," said Verano.

So who was this powerful woman? Experts are researching that question. She was obviously of very high status, says anthropologist Christopher Donnan said. But for now, "she's an unknown character."

See page 53.

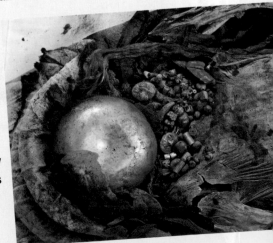

A golden bowl covers the face of a mummy discovered in a pyramid in Peru. Scientists believe this mummified woman may have been a Moche queen. The Moche lived in Peru from around AD 100 to 800.

47

# Digging Up the Past

**Have a look at the tools and equipment used by archeologists at a dig.**

## GETTING READY TO DIG

What does an archeologist do first when she gets to a dig site? She turns the site into a grid that looks sort of like a giant piece of graph paper. Archeologists call this "gridding a site."

The archeologist creates a grid of equal-sized squares on the ground. Then she gives each square its own number.

Next, she copies this grid onto a piece of graph paper. Each tiny square on the paper represents a square on the ground.

When an archeologist finds an artifact, she labels it with the number of the square in which it was found. She also goes to her graph paper and makes a note showing where this artifact was found.

Later, the archeologist can consult her graph paper and know exactly which artifact was found where. Also, archeologists in the future can consult these grids to review the history of the dig.

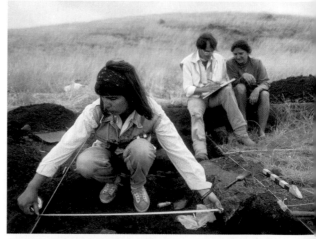

An archeologist starts a grid on a dig on Easter Island. To make this grid, she's using measuring tape, string, and wooden stakes.

# EXCAVATING

**trowel** This is the most common tool on an excavation site. It is used to slowly and carefully remove dirt, one layer at a time.

**shovels and buckets** Archeologists use shovels and buckets to remove large amounts of dirt. They are used only when there aren't many artifacts in the area.

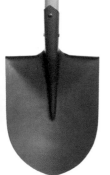

**brush, dental pick, spoon, and dustpan** These are used to excavate small objects.

**screens** Screens like this one are used to sift dirt that's been removed from the site. They catch small objects.

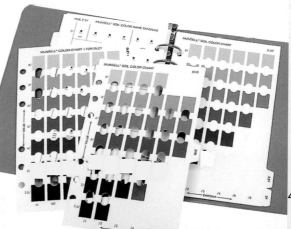

**Munsell book** This book shows the colors of different kinds of soil. Archeologists use it to note the color of the soil where the object is found.

# RECORDING THE WORK

**pen, notebook, and camera**
Scientists use these to record what is found at the site. Archeologists must keep exact records. Once something is taken out of the ground, you can't re-create how it was found!

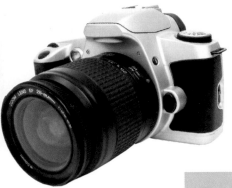

**ruler and graph paper** These are used to make detailed maps of sites.

# BACK IN THE LAB

**toothbrushes** They are used to brush dirt off of objects.

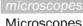

**microscopes**
Microscopes are used to take an even closer look at things.

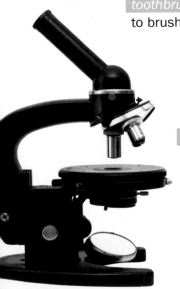

**rulers and scales** Every object that is found must be measured and weighed.

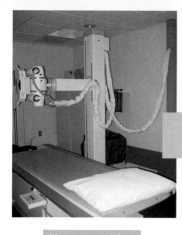

# HOW OLD IS IT?

## How do archeologists know how old artifacts are?

*X-ray machine*
These machines use radiation to take photos of the organs and bones inside a body.

Archeologists talk about "dating" the objects they find. There are two kinds of dating.

*CT scanner* A CT scanner creates a three-dimensional X-ray of the inside of the body. CT stands for *computed tomography*.

**Absolute dating** uses scientific tests to figure out how old the object is. One of these tests is carbon dating. Carbon dating is a way to find out the age of things that were once living. This technique was developed in the 1940s. Scientists realized that measuring the amount of radioactive carbon left in an object that was once alive can give information about how old the object is.

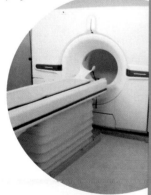

**Relative dating** places the object at a certain point in time. For example, if you dig up your backyard, you may find an old hubcap. If you keep digging, you may find a broken lamp. The lamp is deeper in the ground, which may mean that it was used before the hubcap.

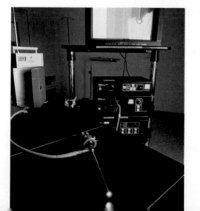

*endoscope* This is a long, thin tube with a small camera on one end. It can be inserted into a body in order to look at organs, bones, and joints.

# HELP WANTED:
# Archeologist and Anthropologist

**24/7: How did you become interested in archeology?**

**DR. SARAH WISSEMAN:** I went on a program in Israel after my freshman year in college. It offered a month of classes and a month digging at a site. I was completely hooked. I loved the fact that you can't sink a spade anywhere in that country without turning up something ancient.

**24/7: What was your education?**

**DR. WISSEMAN:** I got an undergraduate degree in anthropology. Then I got my master's and PhD degrees in classical and Near Eastern archeology. I started taking Greek and Roman classes, and I was invited on a dig near Siena, Italy.

**24/7: How did you get interested in mummies?**

**DR. WISSEMAN:** Back in the early 1990s, I got a phone call from the Spurlock Museum [in Illinois]. They said, we have a mummy, and you can have nine months to examine it. But you can't cut it open because we have to put it on display.

[We used CT scans to examine] the skeleton and organs. Before we had this technology, it wasn't possible to see what was inside a mummy without sawing it open.

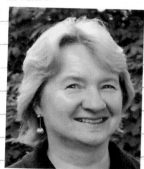

Dr. Sarah Wisseman is the director of the Program on Ancient Technologies and Archeological Materials at the University of Illinois at Urbana-Champaign.

See page 47.

# Q&A: DR. JOHN VERANO

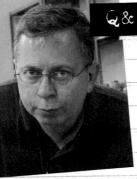

Dr. John Verano is a professor of anthropology at Tulane University.

**24/7:** Recently, you worked with a mummy of a woman warrior found in Peru. What was your role?

**DR. JOHN VERANO:** I went to Peru when they were ready to take [the mummy] out of the ground. I observed as they unwrapped the body in the lab. It took two months. It was a very complicated mummy. There were several bundles wrapped one inside the other with hundreds of yards of cotton.

**24/7:** The mummy of the woman warrior was buried with war clubs and jewelry. Why?

**DR. VERANO:** War clubs could be symbols of power. Or it could be that [people] gave her weapons for protection in the afterlife. She also has a necklace of human heads made in gold. Might these symbolize the heads of enemies taken in battle? We think she was high-ranking because of all the beautiful objects buried with her and because she was buried near the top of a pyramid.

**24/7:** What else was interesting about this mummy?

**DR. VERANO:** She had tattoos. They are mostly geometric designs on her left arm. There are spiders, crabs, worms, and mythical creatures on her right arm.

**24/7:** So what kind of person makes a good archeologist?

**DR. VERANO:** Someone with an interest in adventure and travel, who doesn't mind roughing it at times. You also need to be calm, patient, and able to concentrate. You also need a sense of curiosity, a willingness to do something different—and the good sense to use sunscreen!

# DO YOU HAVE WHAT IT TAKES?

## Take this totally unscientific quiz to see if being an archeologist might be a good career for you.

**1** **Do you pay attention to detail?**
a) Yes. I notice everything, no matter how small.
b) Only if I'm really interested in the subject.
c) I don't notice a thing.

**2** **Are you organized?**
a) Yes. I file all my class notes, and I color code my calendar.
b) I'm organized in some areas, but others are a disaster!
c) No. I'm constantly losing my keys, my favorite sneakers, my notes.

**3** **Are you interested in traveling to foreign places?**
a) Yes. I read articles and books about other countries.
b) Sometimes. But it makes me nervous.
c) No. I'd much rather work in an office every day.

**4** **Do you like to learn about different people's customs and ways of living?**
a) Yes. I like reading and finding out how people lived in the past.
b) I like learning about other ways of life, but I'm most comfortable with what I'm used to.
c) No, I pretty much think my way of life is the best way.

**5** **Are you willing to rough it if you have to?**
a) Sure! Sleeping in a tent, cooking over a campfire, and swatting mosquitos sounds like a great day to me!
b) I can do it, but I'd want to get to a hotel after a while.
c) No way. Indoor plumbing and air-conditioning are crucial for me.

### YOUR SCORE

Give yourself 3 points for every "a" you chose.
Give yourself 2 points for every "b" you chose.
Give yourself 1 point for every "c" you chose.

If you got **13–15 points**, get out your trowel!
If you got **10–12 points**, volunteer to work on a dig or at a museum and see how you like it.
If you got **5–9 points**, archeology may not be right for you. But keep looking until you find the perfect career!

# HOW TO GET STARTED...NOW!

## GET AN EDUCATION!
▶ In high school, focus on developing basic skills, such as math, science, English, and history. Archeologists spend a lot of time writing papers, and they use math to analyze their findings. It's also useful to study a foreign language and learn computing skills.

▶ Get a college degree. Most colleges offer degrees in anthropology, with classes in archeology. However, if you want to be an archeologist, you need to get at least a master's degree in anthropology. You also have to work on archeology projects.

## VOLUNTEER!
Several organizations offer middle school and high school students a chance to take part in archeology digs. Go to page 56 for Web sites with more information on volunteer opportunities.

## LEARN WHO'S HIRING!
The bad news is that it's not easy to get a job at a college, university, or museum. There aren't many openings, and lots of people want those jobs.

The good news is that there are a lot of jobs in other areas. Here are some of them.

## It's never too early to start working toward your goals.

▶ **State Governments:** Every state has a State History Preservation Office that employs one or more archeologists.

▶ **U.S. Government:** There are archeologists working for the U.S. Forest Service, National Park Service, Bureau of Land Management, and the U.S. Army Corps of Engineers.

▶ **Private companies:** They hire archeologists to excavate archeological sites before they're destroyed by construction projects.

## BUT WHAT ABOUT THE MONEY?
▶ Your salary will depend on your level of education, years of experience, and employer.

▶ A field assistant with an undergraduate degree may earn $10 to $12 an hour.

▶ A college professor or museum director may earn $80,00 to $100,000 a year.

▶ An average salary for someone in between—such as an archeologist with an advanced degree and several years of experience—is $45,000.

# Resources

**Looking for more information about mummies?
Here are some resources you don't want to miss!**

## PROFESSIONAL ORGANIZATIONS

### American Anthropological Association
www.aaanet.org/index.htm
2200 Wilson Blvd Ste 600
Arlington, VA 22201-3357
**PHONE:** 703-528-1902

Learn about the research at one of the biggest anthropology centers in the country!

### Archaeological Institute of America
www.archaeological.org
656 Beacon Street, 4th Floor
Boston, MA 02215-2006
**PHONE:** 617-353-9361
**E-MAIL:** aia@aia.bu.edu

This is America's oldest and largest organization devoted to the world of archeology.

### Society for American Archaeology
www.saa.org
900 Second Street NE #12
Washington, DC 20002-3560
**PHONE:** 202-789-8200
**E-MAIL:** headquarters@saa.org

Archeological resources are available on this Web site.

### Canadian Archeological Association
www.canadianarchaeology.com
Royal Saskatchewan Museum
2445 Albert Street
Regina, SK S4P 3V7
**PHONE:** 306-787-2815

This is Canada's foremost archeological center, which is at the cutting-edge in the field.

### Canadian Association for Physical Anthropology
www.utsc.utoronto.ca/~chan/capa/
Department of Anthropology
The University of Western Ontario
London, ON N6A 5C2

Learn about the archeological research taking place throughout Canada.

### Society for Historical Archaeology
www.sha.org
15245 Shady Grove Road, Ste. 130
Rockville, MD 20850
**PHONE:** 301-990-2454
**E-MAIL:** hq@sha.org

Learn more about educational and career training opportunities in archeology.

# WEB SITES

## The Animal Mummy Project in the Cairo Museum
www.animalmummies.com

The Cairo Museum has the largest collection of animal mummies in the world. This site covers how the animal mummies have been studied, what has been learned about them, and how the mummies are conserved.

## The Archaeology Channel
www.archaeologychannel.org

Check out the streaming videos on this site, which showcase archeological projects from around the world.

## Dig Magazine
http://digonsite.com/

This is the Web site of Dig magazine, the archeology magazine for kids. It includes a useful state-by-state guide to archeological events.

## National Association of State Archaeologists
www.uiowa.edu/~osa/nasa/

This Web site offers a directory of links to state archeological organizations.

## NOVA: Mysterious Mummies of China
www.pbs.org/wgbh/nova/chinamum/

This is the Web site for the NOVA TV special on the Caucasian mummies in China.

## NOVA: The Perfect Corpse
www.pbs.org/wgbh/nova/bog/iron-nf.html

This site offers a lot of information about bog bodies. It's based on the TV special from NOVA.

## Passport in Time
www.passportintime.com

Get information about archeological volunteer opportunities offered by the U.S. Forest Service.

## Secrets of the Pharaohs
www.pbs.org/wnet/pharaohs

This Web site, based on the PBS series of the same name, offers tons of information about how Egyptian mummies were studied, as well as historical maps and a timeline of the pharaohs' reigns.

## Tutankhamun and the Golden Age of the Pharaohs
www.kingtut.org/home

Learn about the traveling King Tut exhibition, and see whether King Tut is coming to your neighborhood soon!

# BOOKS

Allan, Tony. *Secrets of the Ancient Dead: Deciphering the Past from Tombs, Graves and Mummies.* London: Duncan Baird Publishers, 2004.

Barber, Elizabeth Wayland. *The Mummies of Urumchi.* New York: W. W. Norton and Company, 1999.

Beckett, Ron, and Jerry Conlogue. *Mummy Dearest: How Two Guys in a Potato Chip Truck Changed the Way the Living See the Dead.* Guilford, Conn: The Lyons Press, 2005.

Buell, Janet. *Time Travelers: Bog Bodies.* New York: Henry Holt and Company, 1997.

Deem, James M. *Bodies from the Bog.* Boston: Houghton Mifflin Company, 1998.

Deem, James M. *How to Make a Mummy Talk.* New York: Yearling, 1997.

Getz, David. *Frozen Man.* New York: Henry Holt and Company, 1994.

Prior, Natalie Jane. *The Encyclopedia of Preserved People: Pickled, Frozen, and Mummified Corpses from Around the World.* New York: Random House, 2002.

Reinhard, Johan. *Discovering the Inca Ice Maiden: My Adventures on Ampato.* Washington, D.C.: National Geographic Society, 1998.

Wisseman, Sarah U. *The Virtual Mummy.* Champaign: University of Illinois Press, 2003.

# MOVIES

*Most archeologists don't have adventures like the ones in these movies, but they're still fun to watch!*

**The Indiana Jones Trilogy: *Raiders of the Lost Ark* (1981), *Indiana Jones and the Temple of Doom* (1984), and *Indiana Jones and the Last Crusade* (1989)**

Swashbuckling archeologist Indiana Jones travels the world in search of treasure—and usually finds thrills and danger instead!

**The Mummy Trilogy: *The Mummy* (1999), *The Mummy Returns* (2001), and *The Scorpion King* (2002)**

Ancient mummies come to life and threaten archeologists in 1920s Egypt.

# A

**absolute dating** (AB-suh-loot DAY-teeng) *noun* the use of scientific tests to figure out the age of an object

**amulets** (AM-yoo-lets) *noun* types of jewelry that are supposed to protect the wearer from evil; they were placed on the body and covered with bandages.

**archeologist** (ar-kee-OL-uh-jist) *noun* a person who studies past ways of life

**archeology** (ar-kee-OL-uh-jee) *noun* the study of past ways of life

**artifact** (ART-uh-fakt) *noun* an object, such as a tool, weapon, or ornament, made by human beings

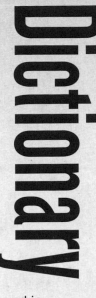

# B

**bacteria** (bak-TEER-ee-ah) *noun* single-celled life-forms found in air, soil, water, and human bodies

**bog** (bawg) *noun* an area of wet, marshy ground

**bog dog** (bog dog) *noun* the preserved body of a dog found in bogs in northern Europe, near where human bog bodies have been found

# C

**canopic jars** (KAN-oh-pik jarz) *noun* jars or vases used by the ancient Egyptians to hold organs during the mummification process

**carbon dating** (KAR-buhn DAY-ting) *noun* a scientific test that figures out the age of an object by measuring the amount of radioactive carbon is left in the object

**Caucasians** (kaw-KAY-zhunz) *noun* light-skinned groups of people, often originating in Europe

**corpses** (KORP-suz) *noun* dead bodies

**cowries** (KOW-reez) *noun* bright shells once used as money

**CT scan** (see-tee skan) *noun* a medical test in which cross-sections of a body are shown on a computer screen; CT stands for *computed tomography.*

# D

**decayed** (dee-KAYD) *adjective* rotted

**dedicated** (DED-uh-KAY-ted) *verb* to have set something apart to honor a god

**DNA** (DEE-en-ay) *noun* a chemical found in almost every cell of your body. It's a blueprint for the way you look and function.

# E

**embalmers** (em-BAWL-murz) *noun* people who embalm, or treat a corpse so that it won't decay

**endoscope** (EN-doh-skope) *noun* a medical instrument consisting of a long tube that is inserted into the body

**excavation** (ex-skah-VAY-shun) *noun* the process of digging up or uncovering something

# F

**forensic** (fuh-REN-zik) *adjective* relating to the use of science to decide questions in criminal matters

# G

**glacier** (GLAY-shur) *noun* a large body of compacted ice and snow that slowly moves

# I

**incision** (in-SIH-zhun) *noun* a cut made usually in surgery

# M

**mummy** (MUH-mee) *noun* a dead body that has been preserved and has lasted a very long time

**mummy gape** (MUH-mee gayp) *noun* mummies often have woven straps around their heads to hold their jaws closed; if that strap is loosened, the mouth falls open, which makes the mummy look surprised. (*Gape* means staring with your mouth open.)

# N

**natron** (NAY-tron) *noun* a salt-like substance

# P

**peat** (peet) *noun* a compacted deposit of partially rotted plant matter

**pharaohs** (FAIR-ohs) *noun* the titles of rulers in ancient Egypt

**preserving** (prih-ZURV-ing) *verb* protecting something so that it doesn't change or decay

# R

**relative dating** (REL-uh-tiv DAY-teeng) *noun* a method of determining whether an object is newer or older than those nearby. Objects found in deeper layers of the earth are typically older than those closer to the surface.

**resin** (REZ-in) *noun* a sticky substance that oozes from pine, balsam, and other trees and plants

**ritual** (RICH-oo-uhl) *noun* a performance of actions in a set way as part of a ceremony

# S

**sarcophagus** (sar-KAH-fuh-guhss) *noun* a stone coffin

**sphagnum** (SFAG-nuhm) *noun* a type of moss that grows on top of bogs and keeps bacteria from growing

# T

**tissues** (TISH–yoo) *noun* body materials in animals or plants

**tomb** (toom) *noun* a grave or room for holding a dead body; in Egypt, tombs were often dug into the side of cliffs.

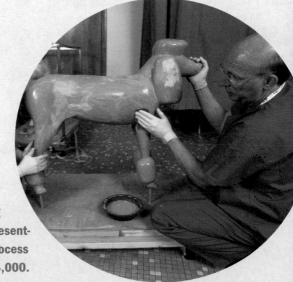

This dog is being mummified in present-day Utah. The process costs at least $4,000.

# Index

**Photographs © 2008:** age fotostock: 4 bottom, 8, 9 (Creatas), 50 bottom right (Emilio Ereza); Alamy Images: 27 (Tibor Bognar), 26 (Kenneth Garrett/Danita Delimont), 50 center (Nikreates), 49 center right (Peter Widmann); AP Images: 33 (Dolkun Kamberi/University of Pennsylvania Museum of Archaeology and Anthropology), 25 (Saedi Press), 5 top, 23 top (Andreas F. Voegelin/Museum of Antiquities Basil); Art Resource, NY: 23 bottom (Werner Forman), 11, 21, 22 (Francois Guenet), 20 (HIP/Ann Ronan Picture Library, London), back cover, 45 center (Erich Lessing), 24 (Réunion des Musée Nationaux); Bridgeman Art Library International Ltd., London/New York/The Illustrated London News Picture Library, London, UK: 19; Corbis Images: 48 (James L. Amos), 4 top, 10 (Bettmann), 6 bottom, 49 center (Jonathan Blair), 46 (Gianni Dagli Orti), 30 (Jeffery Newbury), 5 center, 14, 28 top, 28 bottom, 34, 45 top (Reza/Webistan), 61 (Ted Soqui), 16 (Underwood & Underwood), 1, 2 (Vienna Report Agency/Sygma), 15 (Roger Wood); Courtesy of Glen H. Doran, Florida State University: 41; iStockphoto: 51 center (James Benet), 50 top right (Jane Norton), 50 top left (Micha Strzelecki); Courtesy of John W. Verano: 53; National Geographic Image Collection: 39 bottom, 47 (Ira Block), 32 bottom, 32 top, 32 center (Kenneth Garrett), cover (Todd Gipstein); Photo Researchers, NY: 40, 45 bottom (Eurelios), 51 bottom (James King-Holmes); Reuters: 6 top, 44 top (Ivan Alvarado), 3 (Mariana Bazo), 44 bottom (Werner Nosko); Courtesy of Sarah Wisseman: 52; ShutterStock, Inc.: 50 bottom left (Victor Balabanov), 49 top (Simon Krzic), 51 top (R. J. Lerich), 49 center left (Nikolay Titov); Silkeborg Museum, Denmark: 5 bottom, 35, 36 top, 37, 39 top, 42 top, 42 bottom; X-Rite Incorporated: 49 bottom.

Maps by David Lindroth, Inc.

**A**rcheology is one job where it pays to get your hands dirty! If you're interested in becoming an archeologist, you should read all you can about the field, of course. But hands-on experience is the best way to find out if you'd like the life of an archeologist. Even if you're still in high school, you can work as a volunteer because there are a lot of programs for people who want to explore archeology, either as a job or a hobby.

To find out where you could volunteer, start by going to some of the Web sites listed in the Resources section of this book that starts on page 56. You may be lucky enough to find a dig near your hometown!

If there isn't a nearby volunteer program, try making a list of museums and universities near your home. If the museum has archeological exhibits, call the curator to see if you can volunteer to help out behind the scenes. If the university has an anthropology or archeology department, call the department head to see if any professors have projects that you could work on. If the person you talk to can't help you, ask if he or she has any other ideas about how you could learn more about the field.

Here's another tip: Before you call someone out of the blue, prepare a short account of who you are, why you're calling, and what kind of information you want. And be ready to talk to a few people before you get through to the one who can help you out. Be persistent and be polite—you may end up with a chance to pursue your dream, just by picking up the phone!

Good luck, and keep digging to learn more!

## ACKNOWLEDGMENTS

I would like to thank the following people for their help with this book:

Dr. Victor Mair
Dr. John Verano
Dr. Sarah Wisseman

**CONTENT ADVISER:** Arthur Aufderheide, Pathologist, University of Minnesota-Duluth Medical Center